Secret to Regenerate Your Health for Life

-Yoga & Fitness for Everyone-

By Amaechi Obi

1

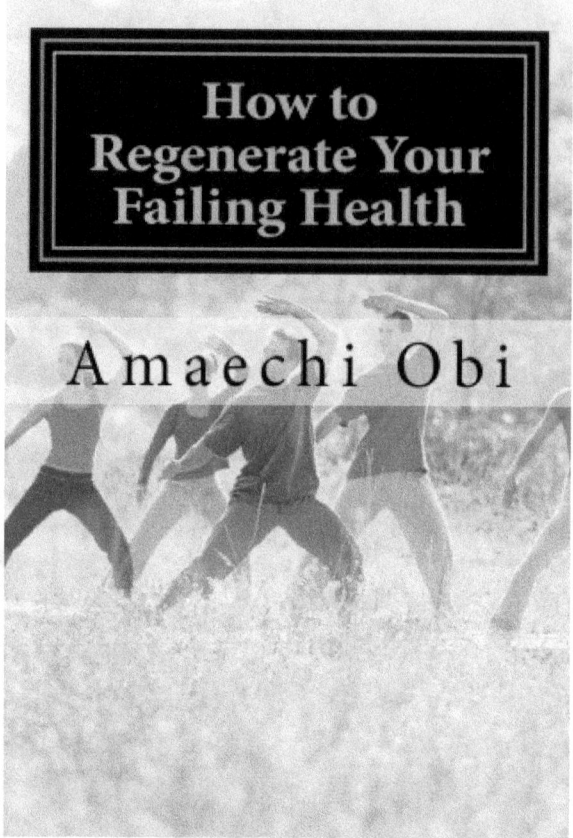

How to Regenerate Your Failing Health

Amaechi Obi

Table of Content

Introduction

Part 1

Part 2

ACTION SEQUENCE TO REGENERATE YOUR DAILY HEALTH

SCENE ONE: SLEEP WELL ALL NIGHT; CONNECT WITH YOUR SUBCONSCIOUS

SCENE TWO: WAKING UP ALL MORNING; STRETCH AND DRINK WATER

SCENE THREE: APPRAISE YOURSELF IN THE MIRROR ALL MORNING

SCENE FOUR: EXERCISE AT WILL; COPY FROM OTHERS

SCENE FIVE: YOGA POSES; PRACTICE AS MUCH AS POSSIBLE

SCENE SIX: TAKE A SHOWER OR BATH ALL MORNING

SCENE SEVEN: **HUG** AND KISS COLLEAGUES WITH WARMTH

SCENE EIGHT: HUG AND KISS OTHERS WITH WARMTH

SCENE NINE: PLAY WITH YOUR KIDS AND FAMILY AT HOME

SCENE TEN: RELAX AS YOU WISH BEFORE BED TIME

PART 3

MY SECRET HEALTH TESTIMONY

INTRODUCTION

To educate others properly, you must have been properly educated in your chosen field. To know something you must seek or ask for it; to have something and make it yours, you must give something greater or equal to that which you ask for.

The above age long proven phrases are the few of the subtle rules of nature, which fortunately or unfortunately lay among the unchangeable rules that govern everything we do, know or have in this world today.

This is not a normal book defining, clarifying, and describing or narrating life's issues as usual: what happened, where, who, when and how. This is a due confession, a live testimony in support of the truthfulness in the "Universal Laws of Nature" and how they affect us positively and negatively in our day-to-day affairs.

What is the first thing you usually do each morning you wake from sleep?

Do you go straight to the toilet to ease yourself? Do you go to the kitchen for coffee or water? On the other hand, do you engage in some quick exercise before you start your daily activities?

Whichever way you usually wake from sleep each morning, this book will help you confirm the best possible choices to boost your energy level the natural way from the moment you wake from your night sleep to the moment you go back to sleep at night time.

As nature's general rule, repeating day-by-day your acquired good and positive habits acts as automatic antidote against ill health, as cure for sadness, depression and as stress control! And when ill health, stress and sadness are put on check, then, your health regenerates automatically.

The best choice of goal for all living beings should be to acquire good health and positive energy on a daily basis. For that, you will need to simply listen to and follow the burning desires of your unconscious mind; harmonize your unconscious mind with the physical reality and you will no longer need a coach to excel in all choices made from within you.

In this book also, you will understand why such subtle feelings as love, peace, harmony and happiness standout as the most vital ingredients in the natural regeneration of human health. In the absence of these pleasant feelings flowing within and out of us, we shall be prone to sickness, pain, hate and disharmony. In this book, you will see live photos and series of videos in action showing how we can naturally boost our given health and happiness from our spiritual mind to our physical body and vice versa!

Chapter 1

HEALTH AND HAPPINESS

Permanent happiness is an attitude; a habit cultivated in space and time through grind. To be truly happy, you must decide to be. When you decide to be happy, you must accept to pay the immutable price of constant sacrifice that goes with it. Before you can be happy, you must be healthy; you must attune your inner mind consciously or subconsciously to healthier habits.

What then are those prices that we need to pay in order to attain good health and happiness?

Health and happiness are byproduct of thoughtfully practicing the following virtues:

- ❖ *Forgiveness*
- ❖ *Fairness*
- ❖ *Justice*
- ❖ *Sharing*

- ❖ *Giving*

- ❖ *Appreciation*

- ❖ *Unconditional love*

- ❖ *Compassion*

- ❖ *Sympathy and positive mental attitude at all time*

Living in line with the above list of mental attitude, you must always feel healthy and happy with yourself, those around you as well as with your immediate environment and going beyond. That sensation rewards you with peace and harmony.

Is there any known thing or emotion for human beings greater than the feeling of: good health, love, peace and harmony? Are these not the basic reason for our entire daily hustle and bustle? You need to give time to and appreciate the abundance of things you already have from childhood to this day. You will be healthy and happy. Appreciate! Appreciation increases the feeling of abundance, which is rewarded with good health, self-confidence and peace.

How many of us can keep the above quality for long without fault? Everyone seeks happiness, but, how many of us truly are happy? In addition, why are we not?
Search your minds for possible reasons or answers why you are simply not happy.
Why you are not naturally enthusiastic and optimistic about the life that is freely given?

A happy personality is usually a healthy individual. Happiness requires acts nourished through dedication to pleasant deeds. That is one simple reason many of us cannot afford to be healthy and consequently happy enough to make it a permanent habit. You need not much to be healthy and happy other than you and yourself alone; your decisions, choices and actions.

CHAPTER 2

ANGER – POTENT VENOM AND ANTIDOTE

Anger is potent venom, but a necessary ingredient of life. Do not always reject anger; just handle it and do what is fair and right according to the golden rules of 'feelings'

Anger can define as – Neuro-chemical prod for action; a signpost indicating the things one partially or fully refuses to accept or such things that fail to rhyme in one's own point of view.

Our inherited and imagined view of right and wrong provokes either joy and acceptance or anger and repulsion.

BENEFITS OF ANGER

1. Anger serves to remind us of things about others, the environment and part of us that need urgent fixing.

2. Anger as well as love helps to straighten up our dear lives

3. Anger helps to move us into immediate action. Every negative or positive action depends on our mental inclination and basic education

4. Be angry with yourself for things you are not doing right. Anger in such cases will help to boost your resolve and determination to get things right now and again

5. Anger, when people do things known to impart and impact negatively whether direct to them, others or the environment is rather a good feeling; the wrong we do now can be paid for tomorrow by others somewhere else

ANTIDOTE FOR ANGER

To overcome anger and curtail its destructive 'venom' or energy, you must choose to do right in line with creational rules, which states as follow: Do not feed your negative anger through desire for vengeance, egoism and such conflicting sensations; neutralize, instead with forgiveness, tolerance, humility and unconditional love for the beauty of things and people!

Anger like love is a very potent energy; if allowed without control and discipline, it becomes destructive. Discipline and manage your anger with justified reasons and feel how that surging anger will ebb and die of starvation, and experience it as love, appreciation and pleasant sense of forgiveness engulf and insulate you from its venom.

To be truly healthy and happy, you need in you a veritable sense of responsibility towards you and all things of creation. It feels good and healthy to be responsible for your every decision and action. This is 'Gran-Via' of positive sensation, health, happiness and harmony.

CHAPTER 3

WHAT IS THE ESSENCE OF LIFE WITHOUT A GOOD HEALTH?

What is the essence of your life without a good and vibrant health? Even when you have labored day and night to acquire all that money and material wealth available in our world; but lack a good and vibrant health which will definitely permit you to enjoy and savor your acquired wealth; what will, in such case be your good story? What should be the testimony of your good achievement in life?

Obviously, living a life without a vibrant and sound health is such an acute pain in the anus!

For the above reason, I have meticulously designed and structured this simple, practical and indispensable book to show you, step-by-step how to cure, improve and maintain your precious given health for the rest of your life!

Know it that, there is no magic-baton or short cut to these practices.

Every day you hunger, eat and drink; in the same way, you urinate, defecate and carry out all other natural life's obligations. As your organs dutifully serve you by carrying out all of the above functions; they also require maintenance to continue to serve you well!

But regrettably, majority of us seem to take these facts for granted; and therefore forget or deliberately ignore to service and maintain the good condition of those given organs which are ceaselessly working day-in and day-out to keep us alive and moving; Why?

Are you among those who will wake up from bed all morning and start their day with cigarette, coffee or breakfast in their mouths, and then, off to work or to any of their other daily chores; most, in frenetic pursuit of money and material aggrandizements at the negative expense of their body and soul maintenance.

The question is what are the good reasons for such inappropriate behavior? How can you justify such a blatant negligence for the only thing that you truly own- which is your- good- self?

Whatever your reason maybe, be it due to laziness, deliberate negligence or sheer ignorance; these short, simple and practical exercises contained in this book will without doubt, help you to correct and balance all of such issues preventing you from taking charge and absolute control of your health!

Your good health, happiness through wise adventure done in harmony with your neighbors and environment is the main essence of all lives, in my view.

Experiment with your life to gain wisdom; sacrifice most comfort to gain experience and good health and then, absolute freedom shall be your compensation.

CHAPTER 4

THE SECRET TO REGENERATE HEALTH

Is there any definite and realistic known secret to regenerate our health without external substances or objects?

Yes, your unconscious mind embodies such secret, listen to it and follow it up to conscious actions. You will discover the immense secret within you to remain healthy and happy!

Good health and happiness have more to do with inward attitude and regular habit than hard work and physical exercise.

Happiness and appreciativeness are usual rewards from doing things out of your unconscious concepts of the conscious realm; doing things out of pondered decisions that harmonizes with the psychic and physical- when the seen and unseen things act in harmony. Such subtle feelings jointly constitute the natural essence of wellness and fitness; in order words- the due secret to regenerate your daily health from all your deeds.

Physical fitness is a derivative of doing things: working, playing, dancing, eating etcetera. Just doing things regularly will reward you with acceptable fitness which goes in proportion with the time you dedicate to whatever you choose to do. Regrettably, you may be fit and well from the outside without being happy and appreciative.

It is realistically hard to have and maintain fitness for long when your regular habit become dominated by such traits as anger, jealousy, avarice, mischief etcetera. Such traits, when dominant in your daily attitude constrict the viaduct of psychic harmony and obscure the pleasant flow of happy feelings. To counter that, learn to agree from within out; make peace with your soul, forgive and forget every offense.

Deep down within your mind lies the potentials for all powers! There are certain known secrets to everything under creation. You are already a secret; your birth, growth and maturity are silent and secret sequences of nature. Knowing and understanding such subtle sequences of nature and creation at large surely will help you to discover the open secret to regenerating your given health.

In other words, regenerating health is equal to knowing how to reach the recess of your mind to receive infinite possibilities that will better and balance your life–sequences at all moments to achieve **'Longer Life immersed in enthusiasm and positive sensations'.** Yes, there are very specific natural sequences to regenerate health!

Deep down within you lies the infinite ability to do and know bits or much of every conceivable thing! Because life itself happens to be an organized process; a systematic process which usually springs from conception, to cradle, growth and death as the end.

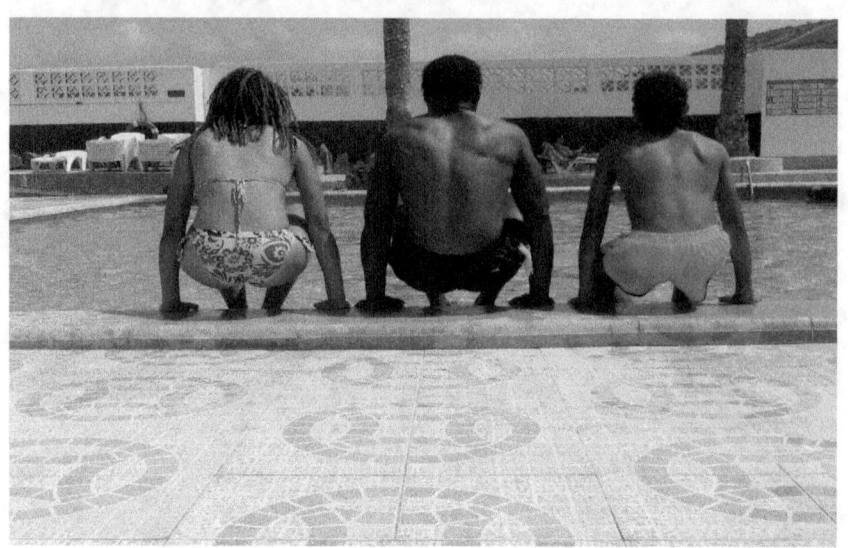

As nature's rule, everything we must do or know carries with it a well-defined process: every sports activity, imagination or knowledge has its naturally endowed process before you can acquire it; even how to eat, talk and walk etcetera. Consequently, at birth, nature has given us the infinite ability to adventure without end, know and experience the abundances of life in its entirety.

Your life is an all-inclusive package with no material cost attached other than the challenges of fact analysis, choice-making, decision taking, action and reaction, which jointly determine how well or how bad you live. You are versatile. You are everything and nothing. Visualize and live your given life in this context and you will be safe.

Chapter 5

YOUR DESTINY IS IN YOUR HANDS

When you say to someone "your destiny is in your hands" what do you actually mean? What do you really want to say or transmit to that person?

If your destiny is in your hands it literally means that your: health, concept, sickness, attitude, happiness and sadness should all be in your hands. It is absolutely true to the best of my knowledge that we can live in sound health with longer life in this world as it is, irrespective of all the calamities and hard challenges looming on us. Once we consciously accept the fact that 'Every Decided Action we take in turn generates undecided Equal Reaction'. In other words, 'Every Sound habit you put up will automatically stimulate sensations beneficial to the body organs and every bad attitude you dish out will also automatically stimulate sensations detrimental to your body organs and of those around you.'

The main secret to regenerate your health is simply based on 'repeating, thinking and reliving such sound and positive habits found generating and encouraging the good feelings being felt by the body's sense organs; on the contrary, rejecting those attitudes noticed generating negative feelings to the body's sense organs.

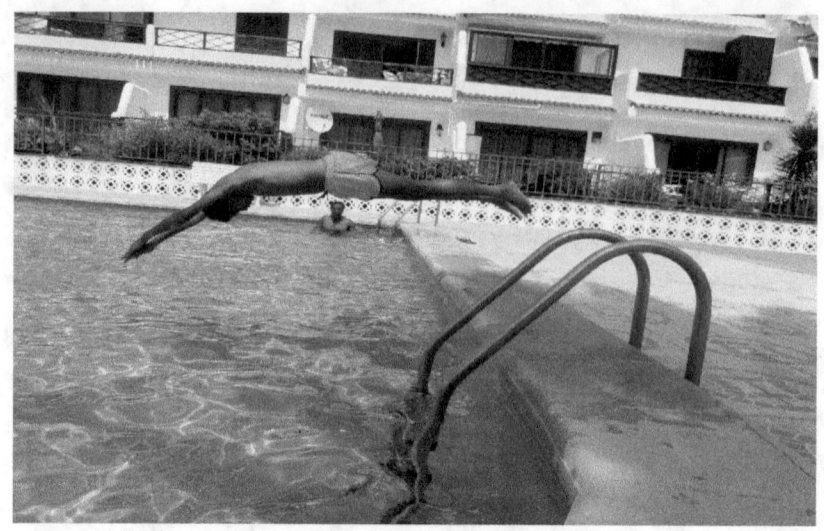

EXAMPLE:

What do you feel when you are: dancing, laughing, playing, or excited about your creativity? The answer is good! You must feel good with the kind of body sensations generated by the above actions without doubt, as far as you are a sane human within our social nomenclature.

Among so many other simple and natural activities, you can adopt to improve your health and happiness: whenever you play, dance, laugh or positively excited; mostly, if not all your body organs benefit from the kind of pleasant sensation generated in relation to the action carried out. Concisely, such is the secret-root to regenerate health and guaranteed long-life in sound sensations.

If you truly desire to live long without much sickness, pain and disillusion all you have got to do now is to start: dancing like crazy; laughing yourself out of breath; playing like a dog and working like an Ant; such are Success Habits. Adopt and attune your mind to them for a year or less. We will want to hear your personal results or testimony. It is all as simple as that! Because, when you do not laugh, play positively and engage consciously in works you choose and enjoy doing, it's hard to feel good and be happy and healthy!

TIPS

The realistic and unbeatable secret to achieve recurring or regenerating-health is to aim to remain a child in mind and in reasoning, metaphorically speaking; do not aim to become an adult under this social standard, doing so will surely reward you with negative and unnecessary stress which will tend to thwarting your endowed positive potentials!

Follow your mind and do not aim to become a socially responsible adult; think as and remain an innocent child; this way, you will have a better chance to live out your days in admirable health; so that doctors, nurses and their drugs will never be your portion!

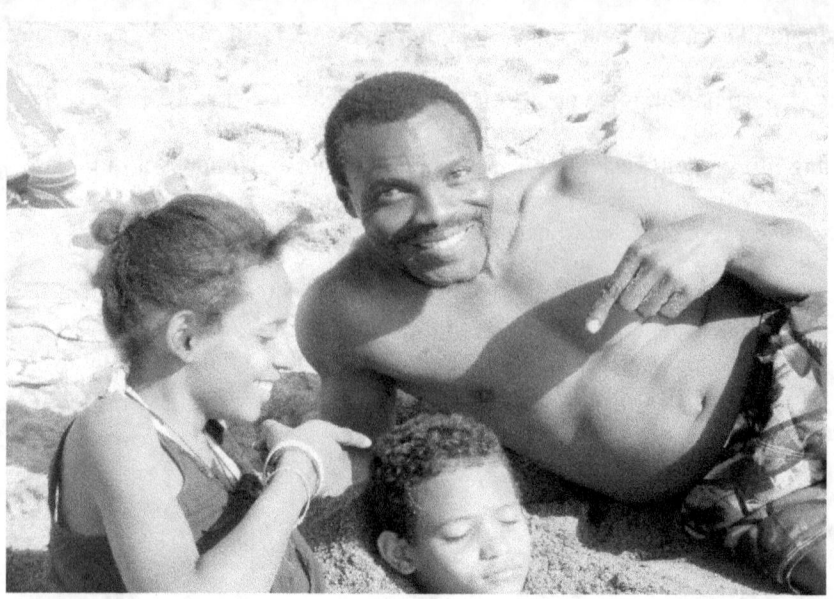

AIM

- ❖ The main aim for this program is to show you with simple and practical examples how to awaken the infinite ability and potentials deep down within you.

- ❖ To empower your use of free imagination, choice and decision to attain a realistic control over your given life; from inside out.

- ❖ To systematically show you the best way to learn about you from inside; and the best possible ways to teach yourself anything you want to know or do, particularly dealing with your state of general wellbeing.

Below is the Ten Regular Scenes of habit you must adopt to have full benefit of this program which kicks off from the moment you go to sleep at night and ends at the moment you go back to sleep to end each day of your given life. Follow it with concentration and open mind.

PART 2

ACTION SEQUENCE TO REGENERATE YOUR DAILY HEALTH

SCENE ONE – *SLEEP WELL ALL NIGHT; CONNECT WITH YOUR UNCONSCIOUS*

From the first day you start this program or lifestyle, choose to begin from early in the morning. So, go to bed at night with this new lifestyle in mind whenever you like, in consideration to your personal routines. Wake up with enthusiasm and with the consciousness that you are going to begin a new way of doing things in your life for a very long time.

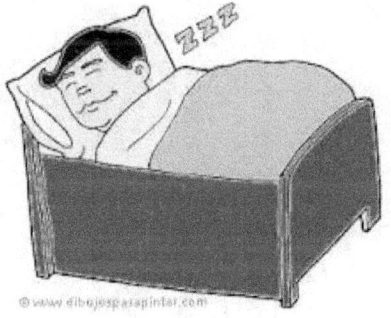

To follow this program effectively, I advise you to buy a Holy Bible or any book that is a motivational/inspirational. In the likes of: Think and Grow Rich by Napoleon Hill; When the Going gets Tough, The Tough gets going by Robert Schuller; Rich dad, Poor dad by Robert Kiyosaki, Holy Koran; etc. You do not have to acquire any of the above books; they are just examples of the kinds of books that can motivate or prod you into positive actions. I use them often. You can find books that prod you to positive actions. That sets

21

your mind into the right frequency to imagine and reflect accurately; to make you live and work with appreciation and gratitude!

SCENE TWO – *WAKING UP ALL MORNING; STRETCH AND DRINK WATER*

Waking up at your own time from sleep every morning, according to your schedules; go to your kitchen for a cup of water and straight to your toilet; especially for those in the cities, living in flats or own houses with comfort of personal toilets. Those others without Toilet facilities at their disposals should improvise whichever way possible and within their means.

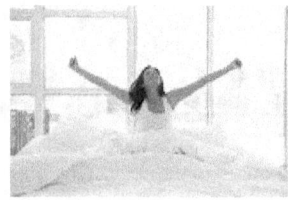

While you sit on your toilet easing yourself, pick any of the inspirational books of your choice, as stated above or other books capable of similar mental and spiritual elevation. Read it carefully as in prayers. Before you start, thank your creator for your life today, show gratitude within you irrespective of what your level of anger, stress and dissatisfaction maybe at that very moment. Be conscious of the fact that you are following a regimented program designed to transform your life to the very best state you have never tasted, felt or witnessed before; therefore, open your mind and do just as I say. You should be your own witness of the proficiency and effectiveness of this program. You should follow it sincerely so that, you can be able to give your positive testimony, when you start to receive the abundant benefits guaranteed with this program for your given efforts!

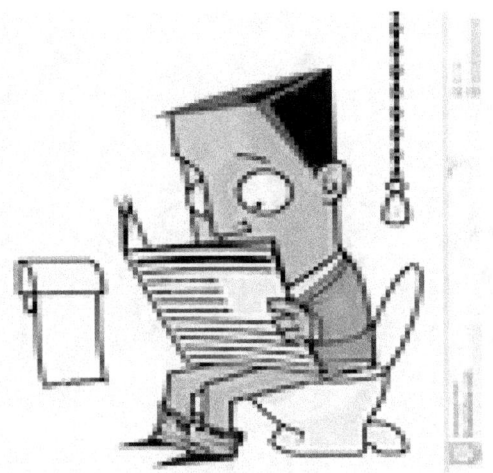

READ WHILE EASING ALL MORNING

You should time yourself before you start with respect to your daily activities: if you have to go to work in the morning or engaged in anything whatsoever, you should be able to conclude the whole exercise within twenty to thirty minutes on a regular basis. If your appointment is at 6 am, for example, try to wake up at 5 am to dedicate at least thirty minutes to recharge your mental and body battery for the day by following this regimen. Learn to wake up an hour before whatever time you should leave your house to attend to any duty. Try to sacrifice whatever necessary all times in order to get what you want for yourself, for your own goodness, wellness and fitness.

SCENE THREE- *APPRAISE YOURSELF IN THE MIRROR ALL MORNING*

-Facing your wall mirror after easing yourself all morning, say it loudly to the wind if you could- "what a beautiful day! Say that from the bottom of your heart, be grateful to the Creator for making you a participant in this glorious adventure - Life" "Thank you, my Father, my Creator for being there silently unshakeable and immutable guiding and watching over me your great son/daughter Amen!

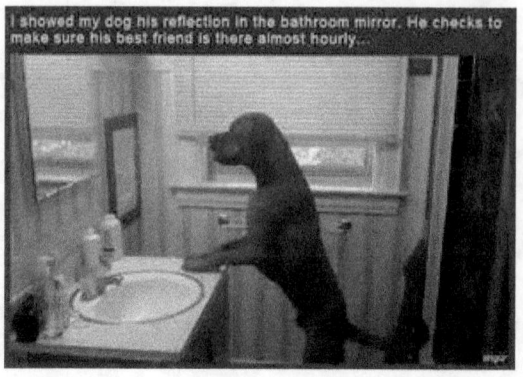

I showed my dog his reflection in the bathroom mirror. He checks to make sure his best friend is there almost hourly...

APPRAISE YOURSELF IN THE MIRROR ALL MORNING

-Facing the mirror, look at yourself direct and deep in the eyes, saying to yourself some positive things like: "I am a nice, great and positive person"; say it with enthusiasm and mean it when you say it! Give yourself a hearty kiss with passion and affection.

-While on that, you should start shaking your entire body slowly; gradually increasing your rhythm and finally with as much vigor as you could summon even for just two minutes; watching and admiring yourself in the mirror as you shake your entire body loose!

The purpose of this kind of activity is to - warm up your blood in order to prepare you morally and enthusiastically for the day's duties ahead; also, to dissipate or wash away some of the cloak or negative energy covering the good and positive spirit, so as to pave the way for a sound and pleasant day about to begin!

SCENE FOUR- *EXERCISE AT WILL; COPY FROM OTHERS*

-If you can and still have the time, make about twenty-thirty counts of pushups. After all that, you will surely notice how your stress and depressive moods will appear to disappear; enthusiasm will set in to take possession of you; and then, everything around will seem more beautiful than you ever imagined! Solution to pending issues will start to arise from the hidden recess of your soul.

PUSH-UP WHENEVER YOU CAN

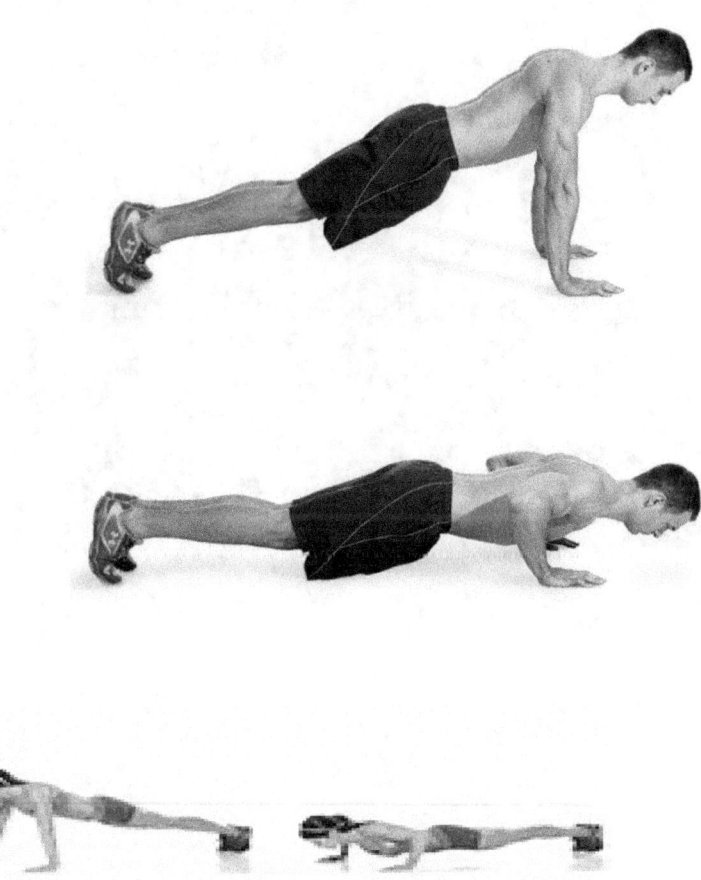

SCENE FIVE

YOGA POSES; PRACTICE AS MUCH AS POSSIBLE

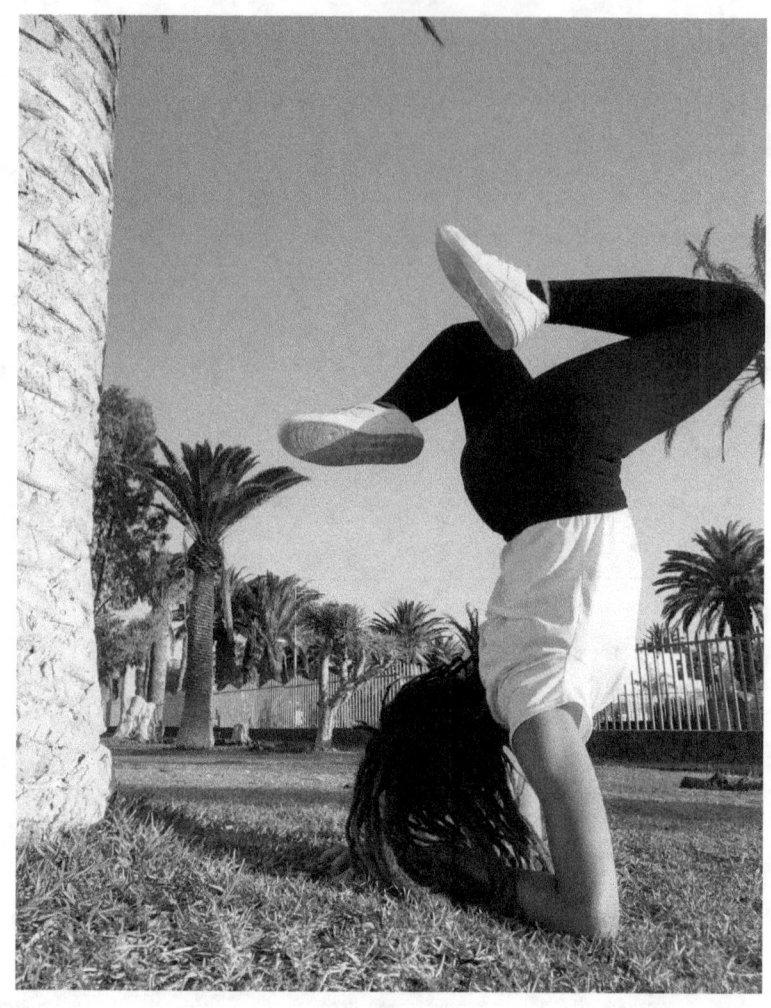

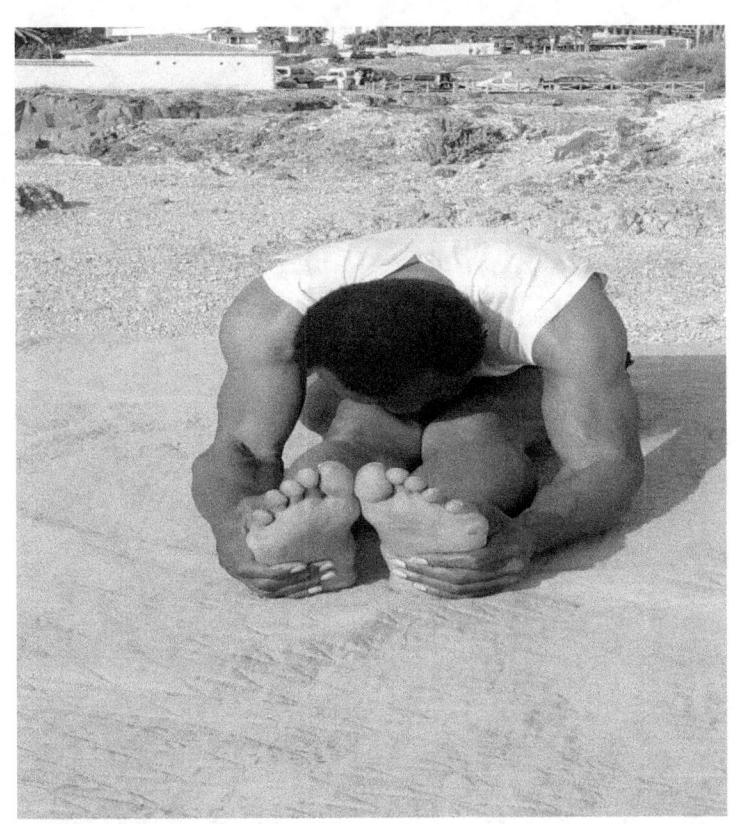

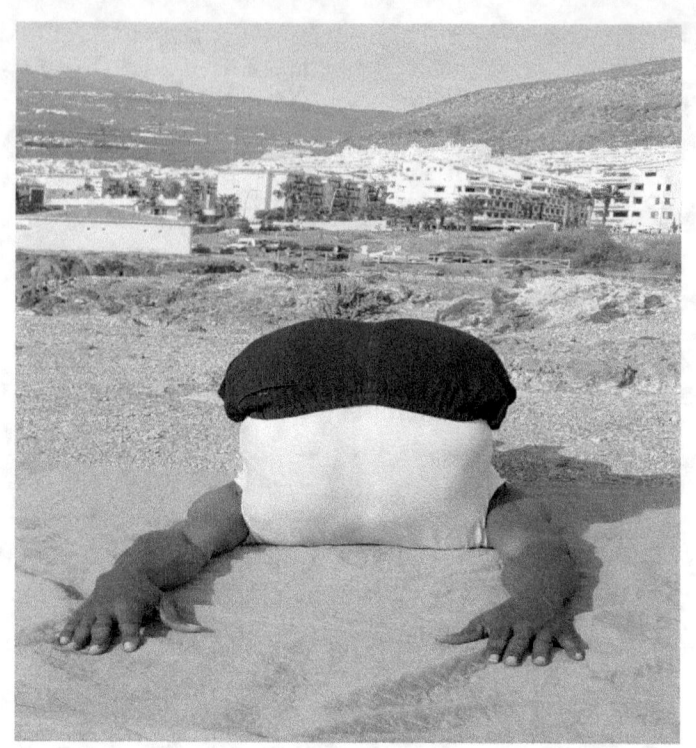

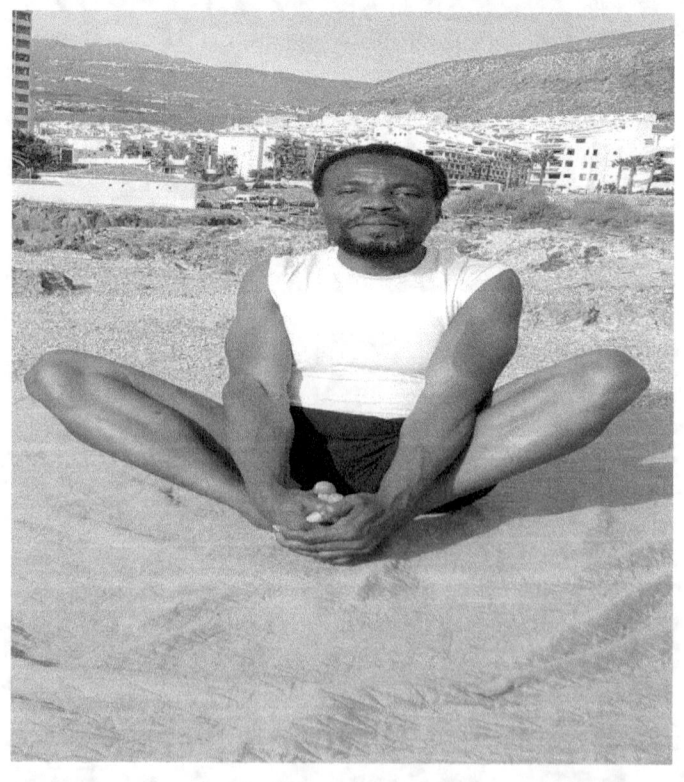

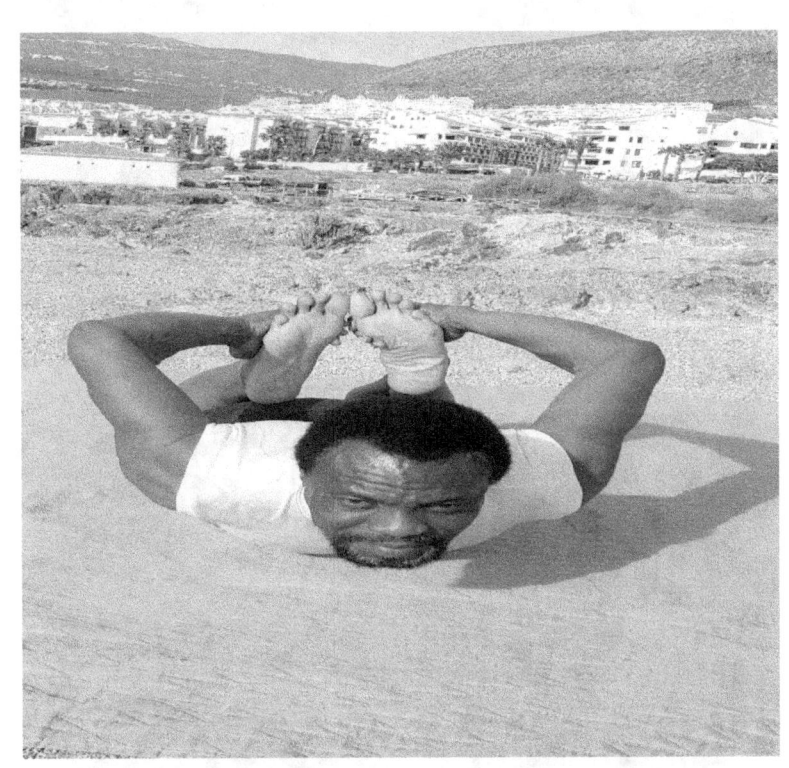

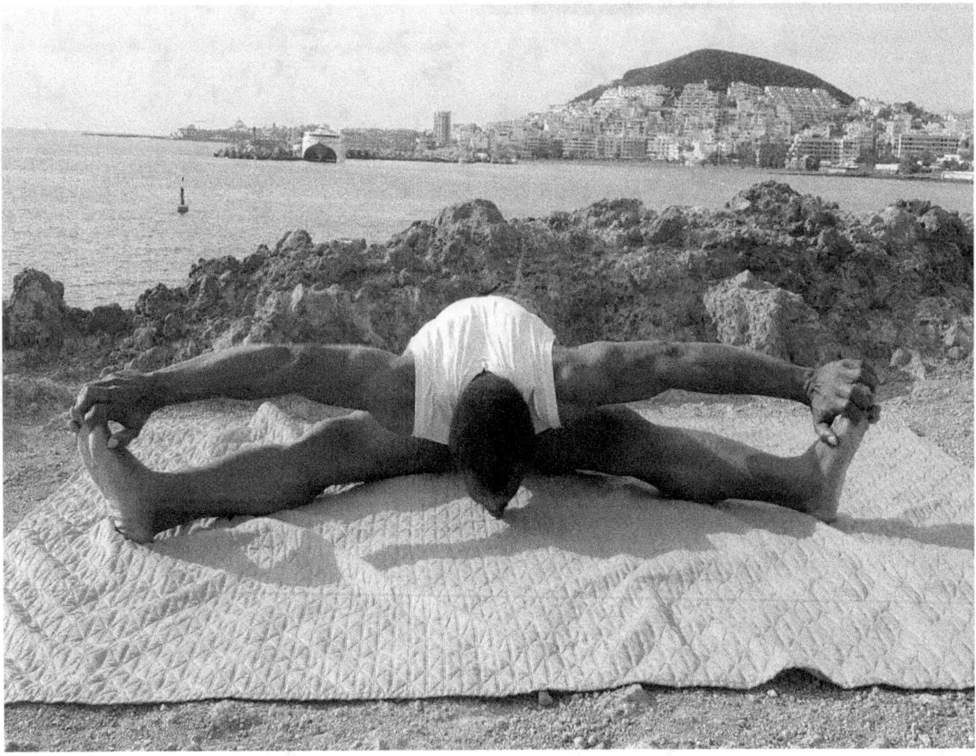

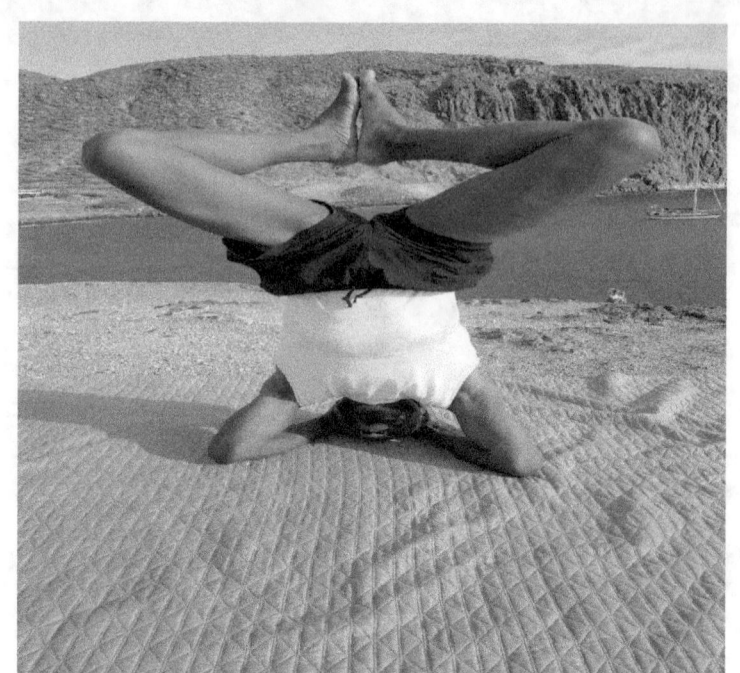

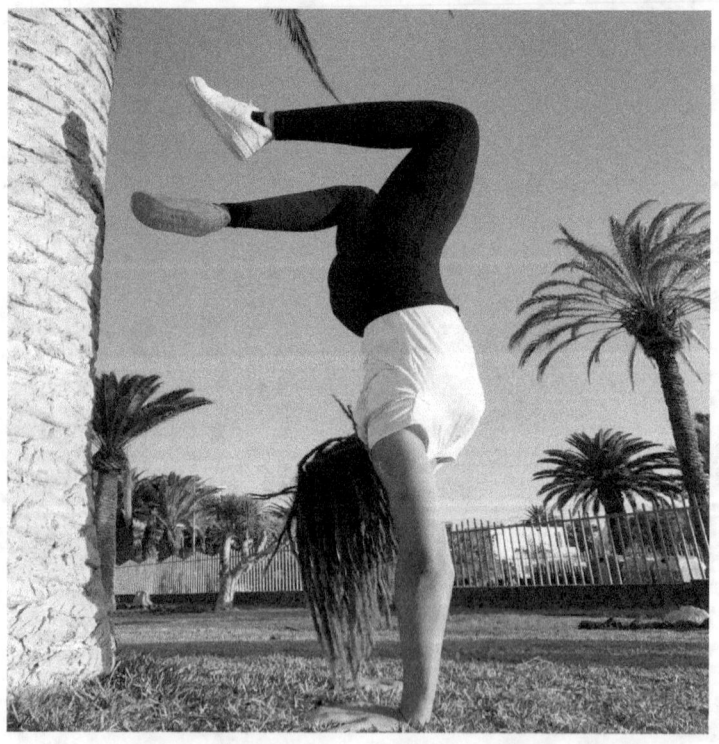

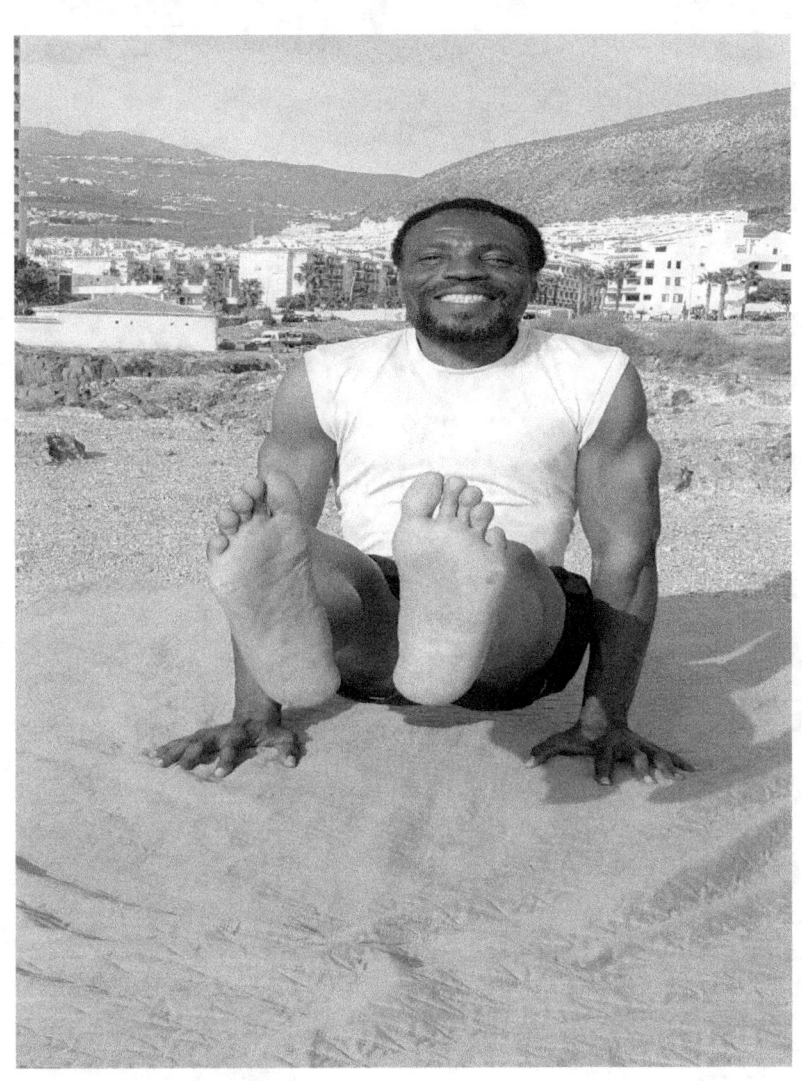

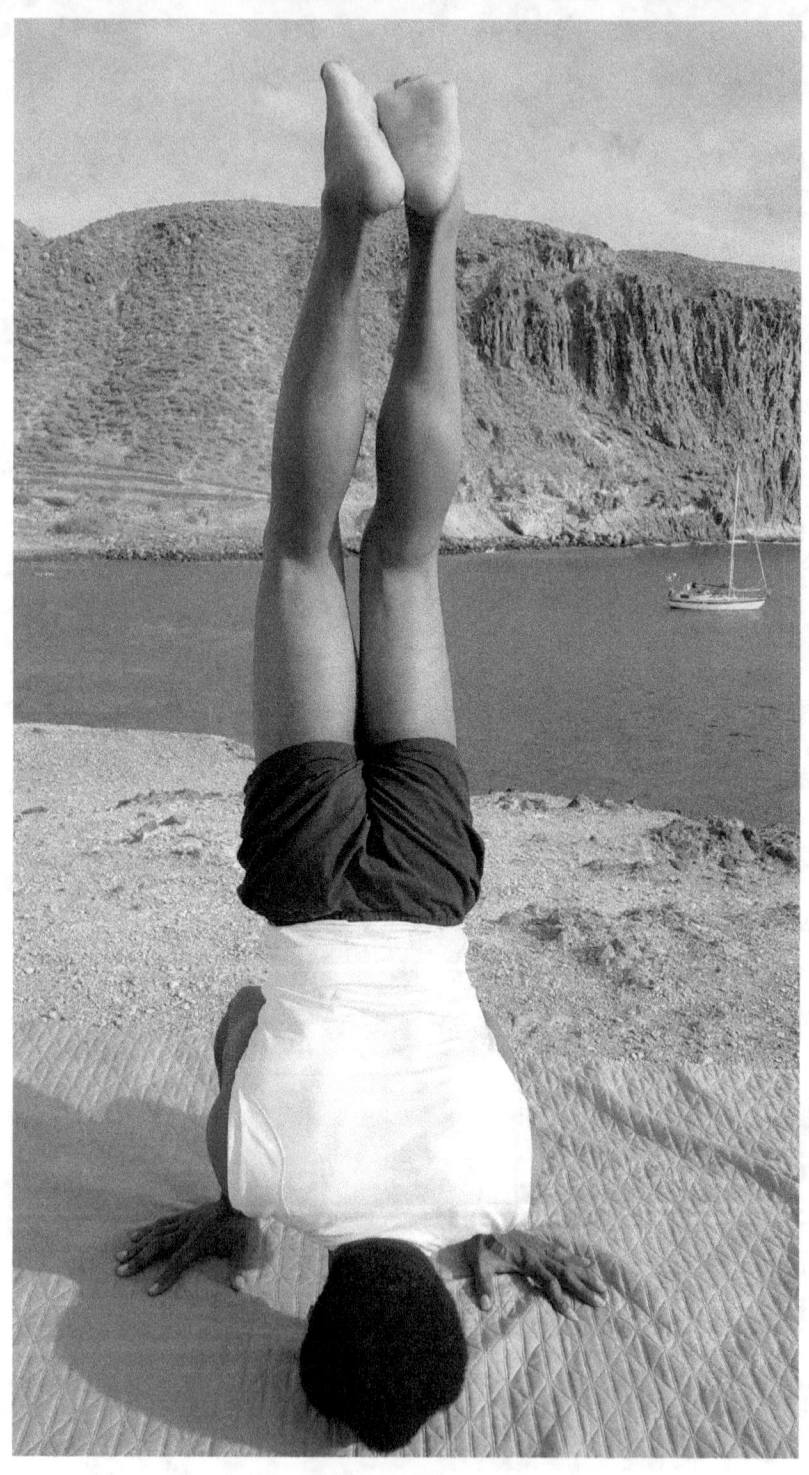

SCENE SIX- *TAKE A SHOWER OR BATH ALL MORNING*

-Take a nice shower with intervals of warm and cold water to make you feel clean and healthy. All these activities will induce in you enough energy and strength to dream, ask and seek with much more enthusiasm and appreciation.

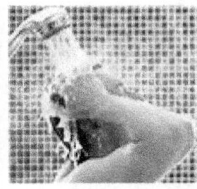

TAKE A SHOWER OR BATH ALL MORNING

-Finally, dress up; have your breakfast and out to work, schools, and others; as you go, share along the way your positive vibrations with all people and things! Show humility, respect and discipline at all moments. With this kind of spirit, you will tend to do everything you want to do with much joy, without expecting rewards; and before long, you will become the 'apple of everyone's eyes and appreciated by all people!

-Remember to kiss your wife/husband, kids, parents; sing your way along and whatever your duty maybe, tackle it with maximum enthusiasm while on it! That is absolute success and freedom!

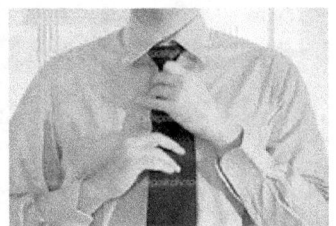

AFTER EACH DAY'S ACTIVITIES -

SCENE SEVEN - *HUG AND KISS COLLEAGUES WITH WARMTH*

As you, finish your daily activities: work, school, sports, etc. Before you leave to go back

home, try to hug your colleagues, kiss or shake them warmly with enthusiasm.

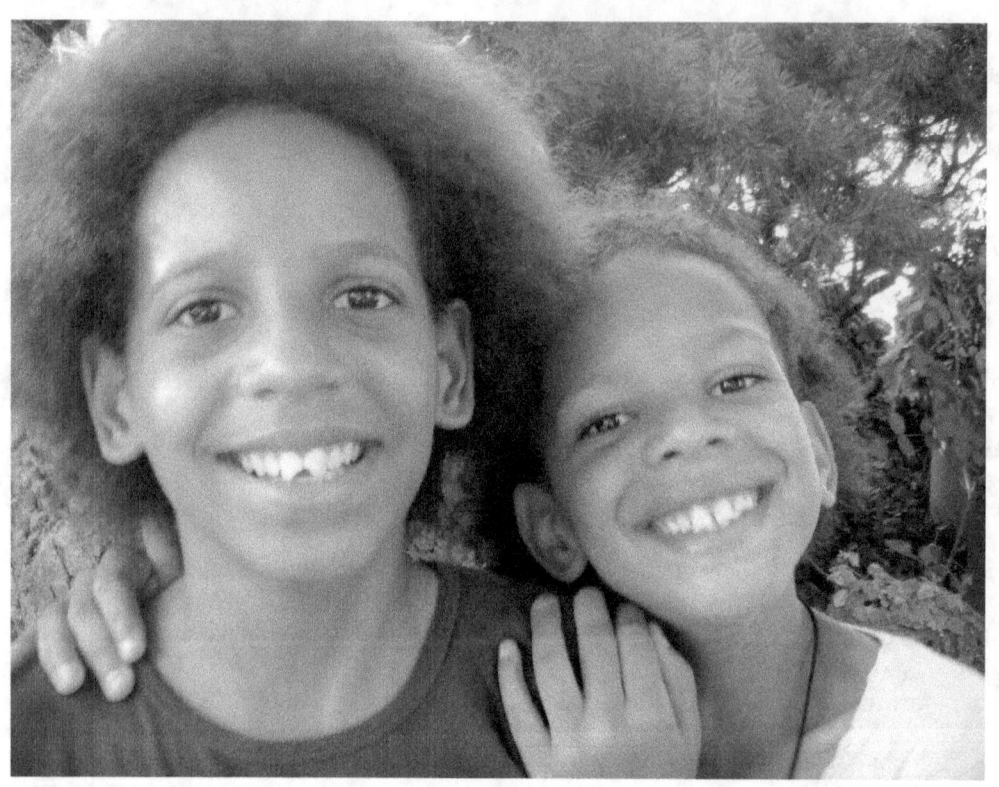

HUG AND KISS WITH WARMTH

SCENE NINE- *PLAY WITH YOUR KIDS AND FAMILY AT HOME*

Reaching home, warmly hug and kiss your family members: wife, husband, kids or parents… then change into 'your happy hour' cloth and then take your family members to your regular spot or sports club. Here you can drink, play, dance with others in joyfulness. Always try to maintain a positive mental attitude at all times - no anger, obscenity, or ugly feelings… these are some of the nature's therapies meant to keep you forever fit and well.

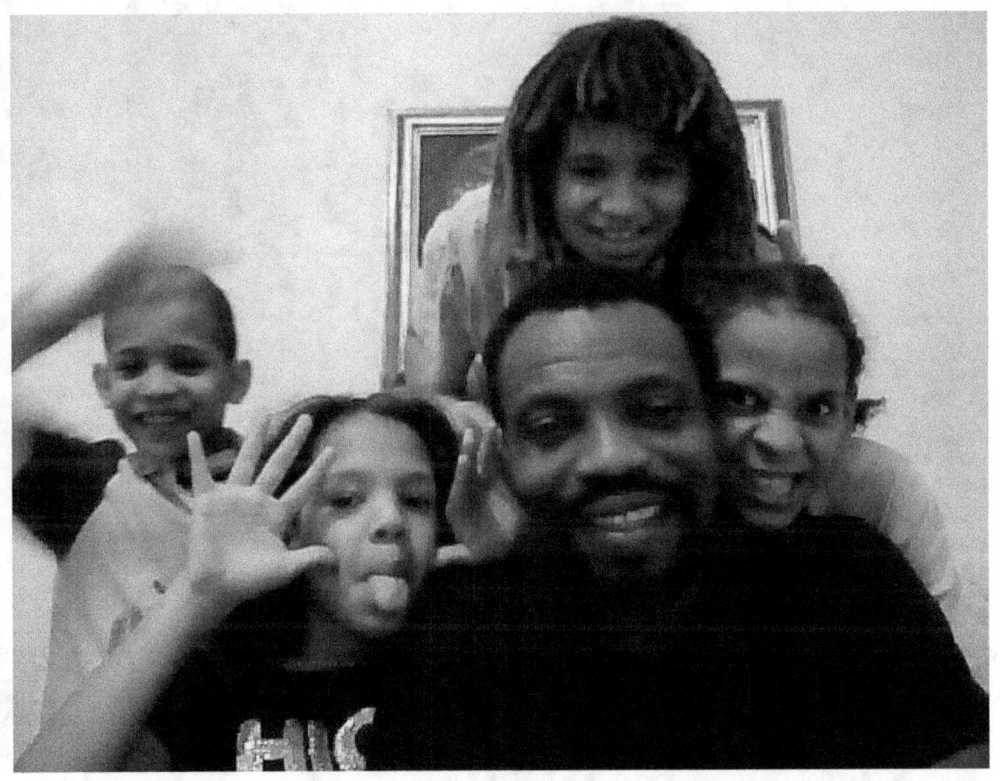

PLAY WITH YOUR KIDS AND FAMILY

Drink reasonably, play reasonably, enjoy reasonably without any form of abuse! Then, go home happy with or to your family for a nice and balanced meal.

SCENE TEN – *RELAX AS YOU WISH BEFORE BED TIME*

Relax and watch a TV, film or what is of interest to you and family; after that, go brush your teeth before you sleep; try to read few chapters of any inspirational book such as the bible and sleep soundly as to wake up for yet another beautiful of a day…

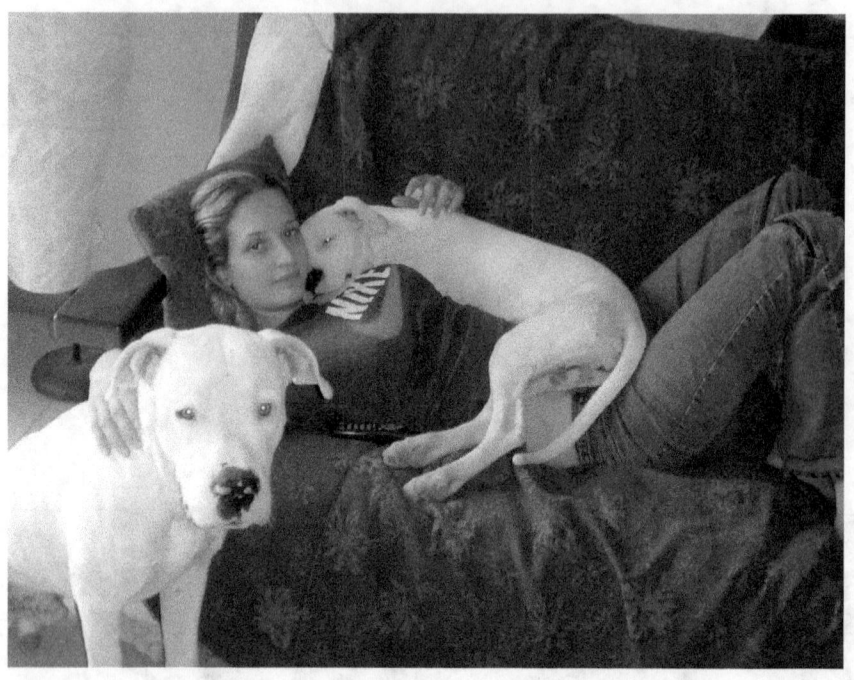

RELAX HOW YOU WISH

This is your routine as a lifestyle for longer period. As you can see, the best things in life are too simple to be true or to seem true! Living your given life with these simple steps will give you the key to an amazing and awesome life!

Congratulations for being among the few to discover and benefit from this unbeatable secret of everlasting wellness-fitness practices!

PART 3

MY SECRET HEALTH TESTIMONY

While a student in India many years ago, I stumbled upon yoga and ever since, it had remained my secret source of out-standing health, wealth and extreme happiness! Yoga discipline since then had unconsciously become my second nature; equal in importance to me as the food that I eat and the air that I breath!

Worthy to note that, I have never officially or privately had neither a face-to-face yoga master, nor coaching lessons, but, however, have always managed to carry along with me different kinds of yoga books everywhere I go. It was my second holy bible! I spent a fortune with joy buying every book of yoga I came across; reading, practicing and verifying with utmost devotion the internal and physical benefits of this unique ancient exercise.

With years of regular practices, I can claim to be a full-blown guru in this discipline and with utmost joy; I want to share my miraculous discoveries with you!

Yoga, when properly and regularly practiced has the hidden potentials to immortalize your body, mind and soul through mental and physical reinvigoration and fortification. For me, the benefits of yoga are equal to none!

My main aim in this short book is not to show you how to just practice yoga, but, to make you know that the blend of basic yoga practices with other fundamental and basic exercises can perform wonders in your dear life; furnishing you with sound health and outstanding wellness you will never have imagined possible.

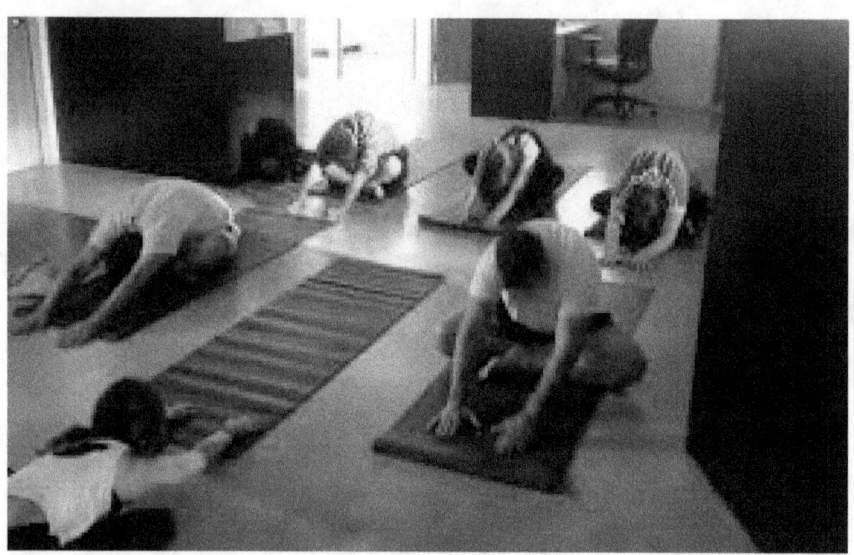

BENEFITS OF YOGA

Yoga exercises alone can deal with and effectively combat many sicknesses that defeat the abilities of many humans. For example, with regular practice of yoga you can combat and defeat such ailments as stress, depression, and obesity; fast aging, wrinkles, blood and lung problems, respiratory and almost everything that may be wrong with your entire body and soul! Then the conscious combinations of other form of exercise do perform the real good-health-wonders, as I will demonstrate to you as we move along.

Most people are not aware that even the simple practice of meditation and correct respiration method can in itself alone deal effectively with depressive moods, high blood pressure and many such illnesses which disturb lots of people; apart from other important health benefits. Lives of many will improve, illnesses will reduce or even totally avoided; and should most of the world citizens learn to manage their health and discipline their given lives appropriately. Doing so will surely give more people the chance to enjoy the awesomeness of excellent living; measured by the standard of good health!

I carefully packaged an interesting, easy and simple fundamental wellness and fitness practices that will not fail to change your lives to the very best once you start this long journey with me. This package is a combination of basic yoga and various other exercises, which will do you many good with minimal stress or hard work! It is ideal for the old, young and children!

You will regain sustainable calm, hope with enthusiasm towards your daily life and day-to-day relationship with your family, neighbors and work colleagues or schoolmates. On daily basis you will be revitalized practicing basic discipline. It is a privilege for you to acquire this package in your health portfolio!

There will be nothing so far that will give you the same advantage and benefit as this package which I had painstakingly prepared for you out of deep love for humanity and for your individual wellbeing. This will surely strengthen your aching muscles once again, and make your life more promising. The benefits cannot be numbered or quantified! As we move along you will undoubtedly testify in affirmation to my claims!

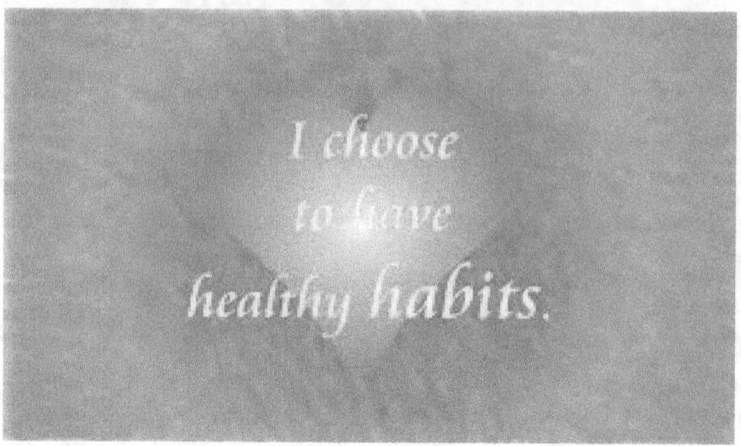

The benefits of yoga to every living body and soul are usually through the sweet sensation it gives to you as you practice regularly. Yoga is a life thing and personal affairs that varies from person to person in accord to individual concepts and mindset. However, for convenience sake, let us just say that on a general basis, yoga can benefit us physically in the following ways:

1. Yoga generates energy, upgrades levels of resistance, concentration and physical forms

2. Yoga practices do not require any special instruments apart from you

3. It helps your body flexibility and free flow of liquid and energy circulation

4. It helps to reduce fat and excess cholesterol.

5. It can be practiced well by everyone: children, man, woman and elderly people.

6. Yoga fixes and betters your physical posture and reduces aging process.

7. It attunes your entire body through adequate blood circulation.

8. It provokes your internal organs, regulates metabolism and suits your endocrine system.

9. Yoga positions can be said to be complete and equilibrated gymnastics.

10. Yoga rejuvenates, reduces tension and shows you how to relax well.

11. It helps you to understand your body better.

12. It helps you to think positively on a long run

MENTAL BENEFITS OF YOGA

❖ Yoga helps you to control emotions, especially angers and annoyances

❖ Gives you a positive and relaxed personality

❖ Makes the mind agile and flexible, therefore, favors free energy flow

❖ Helps to calm the mind and combat stress

❖ It energizes the mind in such a positive way no other exercise does

IMPORTANCE OF RESPIRATION IN YOGA

Correct respiration is the most essential lessons of yoga because it completely helps to control the mind. This is where yoga differs from all other simple physical exercises.

Through the practice of yoga, we have learned that the majority of humanity do not have clue about adequate and proper ways to breathe. Most of us use like one third of our pulmonary capacities while breathing; we apply only the upper part of our lungs! This hardly move our thorax; breathing therefore tends to be fast and superficial; resulting in breathing-in just very small quantity of air into the lungs. This in turn, denies the body organs adequate supply of air necessary for a better functionality.

Good breathing should include the upper part of the lungs, under the clavicles, at the center to expand the thoracic cavity and the lower part. This kind of respiration or breathing that sends more air in the lower part of the lungs is known as- 'abdominal'. This is the best way to supply adequate air to the lower parts of the lungs. It is a slow but complete respiration!

Respiration should be through the nasal cavity- because those hairs in the nose do help to trap particles with germs, dealt with by the mucous. This way the air that travels from the nose down to the lung will heat up with adequate temperature before settling down in our lungs. Mouth respiration losses all those effects and benefits. The length of respiration and expiration is what we use to determine a good yoga effect on the positive note.

OTHER WELLNESS AND FITNESS EXERCISE

The truth is that, to make normal exercise one has no need to worry about deep concentration as in yoga. You can make any form of physical exercise, watching TV, listening to music or at the same time talking and chatting to friends; these are not acceptable while really carrying out yoga practices.

Yoga concentrates on the mental, spiritual and physical balance in harmony, while normal exercises concentrate mostly on the physical resistance and toning of the body organs and muscles. You can make general exercise without really focusing on a particular body organ as against yoga.

If our destiny is in our hands, it then means that everything we need to live well, fit and happy should as well be within us; in our respective hands. In respect, the good and the bad are intertwined; our human duty is to disentangle the strings binding the good with the bad; retain and reuse the good while you flush and reject the bad! As you do this, you will definitely notice the regular upsurge of sweet and pleasant sensation loaded with innermost energy and fortitude.

Everything we do in this life is only to achieve a fruitful life without sickness, negative stress and pain; knowing that made it easy for me to dig and grasp these regenerating health secrets which are intended to create an amazing lifetime discipline which can be readily practiced from wherever you may be now; your social cadre, gender or age.

My Wellness and Fitness Program has no conflict with anything whatsoever! It's a program which had been going through rigorous test for years; meticulously structured to guide you in the proven path leading to absolute health, all through to the rest of your life. This will show you also, a dietary habit that will conform to this kind of discipline. This is an all-round wellness and fitness habit divided into scenes for you to easily assimilate and incorporate them!

Why This Combination of Yoga With Other Fitness Exercises?

Yoga can easily combine along with other forms of fitness practices; it is my intention to show this fact because there are many misconceptions on the subject of Yoga in all cadres of our societies; many believe that yoga is a complete sect of religion on its own. Others believe that, to practice yoga, you must have to know all the yoga doctrines and poses, etc. In this modern world, it becomes nearly impossible to live in such total abstinence as required by the true yogi from the East. For that singular reason, I have considered that majority of people all over the world are deeply engaged with their daily chores that they hardly have time to practice, even the most simple but, essential exercises needed by their bodies to function well.

For the above reasons, I decided to research a bit further and discovered a way that may be easy and convenient for everyone with the least zeal to better their lives without renouncing any of their usual daily activities. Combining the most basic yoga exercises and principles with few normal everyday wellness practices that anyone: old, young and children of all genders can practice daily on a regular basis; and which have the capacity to give you an outstanding wellness and fitness benefits ever put together anywhere!

EXERCISES

MIND AND BODY EXERCISE MUST BE MANDATORY TO ALL-

What is exercise?

Exercise is the act of voluntary or involuntary engagement of body and soul into activities that heats up the muscles and organs causing the heart to accelerate its beat and the blood circulation; this in turn, will help to boost body and soul relaxation as well as; feel of the sense of well-being.

There may not be many people out there, who do not wish to possess an excellent health and the feel of well-being. It is humanly natural for every individual to secretly wish and desire to appear gorgeous, strong and healthy.

However, the big question is how many people in this modern world are able to realize that goal through their personal initiatives without external assistance?

How many people are able to maintain a sound and stable health for so long on a row without any form of external assistance?

How many people understand and believe the fact that everything about their respective health, state of well-being, freedom of all kind and their happiness, solely lie in their hands?

Experiences shows people are not aware of the above facts and few are very much aware of it but reluctant to combine the modern lifestyle with the grind of regular exercises- working in closed offices; sitting behind a computer for hours, or standing on their feet for hours manipulating machines and other such related jobs.

Fact remains that, by the time they leave their respective places of work and get home, they have been beaten by fatigue mostly out of constant routine than of real tiredness.

In few of such cases, some of the people will be willing to make some exercises to subdue the acquired stress and boredom but will unfortunately discover that their inner spirit is not enthusiastic enough to go along with their bodily need. "The body willing but the spirit very weak" as the saying goes!

In all, it feels nice to sit your butt in your swivel chair in front of your Computer (been served and entertained by Microsoft, goggle and the rest) all day working in an office. Nevertheless, the only problem is that type of lifestyle does not help your blood circulation and the enhancement of your body muscles; going on that way for long maybe detrimental to the smooth functioning of your body and soul.

For good health and long life, you must always do things that really sweat or warm your body on daily and regular basis.

Experience shows that nearly all human possesses that secret desires to do their very best for themselves; to be the very best that they could afford to be.

Desires to live long and never to die prematurely and have the very best of all material possession possible that they could afford to have.

Nevertheless, the big question is at the end of the day, how many people do truly realize these goals to their very satisfaction? The proliferation of gyms and spas, hospitals and pharmacies plus places of worship of varying categories is a clear demonstration of that strong inner and secret desire of all to get better and to have the best out of life. However, unfortunately, from the look of things the large number of sick and unhealthy people all around the corner; the large number of people with problem of obesity, anorexics or bulimia; and the large number of people fanatically and devotedly seeking spiritual salvation through prayers at all cost.

Concisely, all of the above clearly shows that "many are truly called but few are truly chosen" as the holy bible said years back!

The above premise, makes the wise to understand that many people do not know enough of themselves because the true meaning of knowing oneself also goes in context with knowing the kind of food that is good for your stomach to digest better for maximum benefit to your entire system.

Entails also, knowing how to gradually nurse your body, your soul, do your daily work, exercise at the same time and keep a positive mind to achieve that secret desire of having the best and being the best that you would like to be and have. These things are the gift of nature for all to possess, there is no magic to it except that of learning to acquire wisdom and keeping a positive mental attitude which harmonizes the forces of nature to make things work out as though with magical sticks.

The good news is, when one learns to understand and control one's mind the eating, playing and working habit will naturally get better. Life will begin to assume a dramatic change toward the possible best– enthusiasm for life and for doing positive things will usually begin to rush back to that person from out of some hidden compartments.

Under such positive mental attitude you will begin to feel that you can do those things that were like impossible to you before, suddenly, you will begin to feel that yes, you can do it and do it right. You will start to train your body and soul according to your own natural pace without need to rely on a coach, weights or any other form of external methods outside of you.

This is one of the ways nature rewards those who appreciate things they already have, and at such a stage, they notice how they will begin to cut down and save on doctor's bills. These things are simple for those who have faith and confidence in themselves; and to them, gradual and positive changes will start to occur in their respective lives in unexpected successions.

TIPS

I have had the chance and the time to practice different sorts of sports and exercises for years ranging from: football also played as a goalkeeper, with a broken finger; those scars will remain with me for life. Games I can play includ: tennis (both table and lawn tennis), basketball, swimming, athletics, boxing, aerobic-dancing, biking, yoga and many more.

I do consider myself a versatile human being; because I am capable of many kinds of sport that I may wish to put my energy in it, no matter how difficult and complicated. Somehow, deep down I am very much aware that nothing is impossible for me to do if I have a cogent reason to do it. In addition, somehow it seems the more I grow in age, the better stronger I become.

Due to my constant kneecap dislocations, I had to give up strenuous exercises such as soccer, goalkeeping (my childhood favorite sport) running and sports that stress the knee. I refused to operate my kneecap injuries because of my mental stubbornness; I always like to run my 'shit' my own way irrespective of the sufferings and loses that may come with it.

As a result, I secretly and gradually began to device other avenues between the abundances of possibilities deep down within me which I kept discovering on daily basis according to needs and desires; sometimes by chance, and other times through mere wishing to try something new; and most of the times through core imaginations and grind.

From all of that, I discovered that the true secret for good health and sound living is never based on becoming Olympic champion in any kind of sport, games or otherwise; in fact, anything done for too long, usually leave some scar behind for the bearer, which others may not be able to see or feel. So, from all these, I found myself deep in the ocean of the secret of good health which I have selfishly and secretly enjoyed for nearly half of my life.

Everyone, especially my close friends used to wonder how I manage to remain so healthy, so athletic. Some use to spy on me to find out if I do practice weight-lifting in secret and many think that way. Why do they think that way? because they will never understand how they could always be busy lifting weight, running and doing all sorts of things to keep fit; and I, instead seem to do 'fuck-all' or nothing but always remain the same in weight, full of smiles, sometimes over enthusiastic and over energetic!.

Today, I want to share those secrets of good health and happy living, which I have secretly enjoyed for nearly well over two decades of my life on this great and awesome world! (You do not know how wonderful this may feel until you begin to apply and benefit from these simple principles). Here are what I was doing- easy and simple; but the trick is on keeping it regular and making it a long-term habit.

MY SECRET LIFE:-

1. Each morning, wake up from bed and head straight to the toilet, (always keep a bible, Koran or any inspirational book permanent in one corner of your toilet) while easing yourself, read even a favorite paragraph from either of those books, as in prayers! Do not wake up and instead head to the kitchen for a cup of coffee, tea or cigarette.

2. When you finish easing yourself, close the book and return it in its place. Do not try to keep reading that book after easing yourself because you have to go to work or have got other things to do- stand in front of your bathroom mirror appraise and admire yourself by reminding your good self how wonderful you are and how wonderful and beautiful this world is. With that, according to your own feeling, your own ways, give thanks and praises to the most high! Prepare your mind to confront this day with much anticipation and enthusiasm!

3. After that, stretch your body in whichever way you are able; for example: swinging your arms slowly, bending your head to your knees over and then standing up straight; sideways and forth; start shaking your body slowly and increasing gradually; then rapidly and vigorously as when running a hundred meters in ten seconds or so. You can repeat this as many times as possible or as your time and ability may permit. (Do not ever try to stress it, be conscious of the fact that you have to go to work and you have to do these things for the rest of your life on earth, and it is targeted to be over in less than ten minutes,

maximum fifteen unless you have more time and wish to push it a little bit longer)

4. Breath hard, even to pant after the body shaking, and then start to breath slowly until you cool off. This is important to warm your blood and permit maximum circulation that washes away stress, depression and many other impurities that may accumulate in your blood system; do this each day even for a minute or two, it will always act as an effective defense against those negative or toxic substances occupying too much space in your body.

5. While doing all of the above, keep admiring yourself in the mirror and be conscious of time because others have to use the restroom as well; you have to hurry up to go to work; which means, you have to wake up at least an extra thirty minutes before the usual time you are used to waking up on a normal day-that should form part of your daily routine. This exercise is to prepare and clean your body for the day's work ahead.

6. If time permit you, add about ten to twenty 'push-ups' even if it just five. That's the way for some years. With time you will naturally increase the number of times you push-up, this is not important, what is important is to keep it regular for years that is where the trick lies. The idea and the motivation is what is important, because that triggers certain positive hormones that performs the

miracle like in little drops of water which can form a river if allowed to drop for years!

7. While in all that, concentrate and imagine a great day ahead of you, imagine a great health and energy accumulating in you. Now start to rinse your mouth and wash your face. You are ready to go to the kitchen for breakfast. You may choose to shower before or after breakfast, the choice is yours – mind you taking a bath in the morning form part of this therapy. Most people especially in advanced countries of the world have adopted that ugly habit of not taking bath regularly due to one reason or the other. However, my advice is, that having a bath whether hot or cold is a way to activate your energy and motivate your morals and enthusiasm for work and for life on day-to-day basis.

8. Do not leave what you can do today for tomorrow; tomorrow is entirely another day. When you live your life this way you permit enough toxins which can manifest in forms that maybe very strange even for some acclaimed physicians to predict due to the fact that this world we live in is run by certain natural or cosmic rules. So, always try to give in your best every day and leave the rest for God or for the creator to rectify!

9. After your bathe and breakfast, you are then ready to go to work or for other activity, you are supposed to be engaged in; with your blood warm and your heart beating rhythmically, your enthusiasm will be on the rise. In this way, you

can work with joy and able to go the extra mile in whichever thing you find yourself doing after wards.

10. It is a crime against God and humanity for any healthy man or woman to have nothing to be engaging his or her energy. (work here does not mean only economic engagements, but rather any form of proactive functions and creativity which will help to enrich yourself or other people around you; not that you are not allowed to do other activities to keep yourselves fit according choice and desires).

These exercises are to show you my personal secret to good health and happiness. It is meant only to activate and warm your body every morning considering the hectic lifestyle of work and time schedule available to the present-day-humanity; this health practices will help you in all ways if kept regular; to boost your daily moral and to fight against depression that comes mostly from daily work routines or inactivity for long.

I usually try to keep my exercise within the span of twenty to thirty minutes irrespective of how busy I may claim to be. I believe we owe ourselves at least that little time in a whole day for every day considering that, without a sound health, life rather becomes an impressive torture instead of the marvelous paradise it should be!

BENEFITS AND ADVANTAGES

-When you are able to practice living as stipulated above, your body and soul tend to be in constant harmony with each other and you will naturally tend to be able to share and communicate with others.

-You will notice that life will begin to have more meanings to you, always full of enthusiasm, which is the basic ingredient of life. In addition, you will be ready to spread relief to anyone anytime and everywhere you may find yourself.

-Your muscles are always relaxed strong and firmly while your skin will begin to look brighter and resilient.

-Your faith in all things both in yourself and in your confidence will all seem to be firmly intensified.

-Fears of the future are removed and your belief in a particular goal is seen more clearly and within arm's length'.

-Your body weight will automatically tend to stabilize in a way that will be suitable to your heart desires.

-You become discouraged from addictions in weight lifting and athletics. You can only do those for fun and pleasure but no more as a form of keeping fit because you will know or discover that you have found a much more convenient and sure way of keeping fit for the rest of your life with little or no stress!

-You will become glad to be giving much more time to your good self because you are now in love with yourself. You will naturally have the feeling to know more of yourself and that is good enough for you on the long run!

-You will discover for yourself that it is not all the great food you eat that gives you ideal health with physical and psychological fitness but, rather, how well or positive you reason that does the magic!

-You will no longer need to neither sleep minimum of eight hours nor need to eat three square meals daily to be sound and healthy!

-Your face somehow will always wear a 'contagious smile' in any situation- even in the face of adversity and unforeseen difficulties!

-And finally, but not the least, old age will cease to be horrible and unfriendly but, this time, likeable and acceptable!

The surest way to obtain all the benefits from this program is only through discipline; a gradual process of understanding of oneself – that very knowledge or wisdom gained within this period is the surety that will give the mind that stability that will never fail to put all things for you into their rightful perspective, health wise and other wise.

We must by now, at this very level of highest technological era, coupled with economic and material boom, come to the stark reality that, if there is no Godly discipline for the lives we deliberately choose to live and for things we do and for how we do them, there will be no easier gateway. This is because, if money and material possession where enough to make us healthy and happy, I guess, over eighty percent of the world population today would have being happy and healthy; and probably even live hundred years and above on the average!

It will be advisable if we can take more seriously some of those seeming minor things of life and always try to put them into consideration irrespective of their seeming simplicity: laughing; assume and accept laughter as a very serious thing of necessity.
Do not fight tears to drop from your eyes whenever you can have the chance to be positively emotional as in laughing and in crying; positive thinking and actions.
Consider all others around you with love and respect instead of with hate and intolerance.

Those are just little tips among millions, through which each individual can utilize to find their pathway towards the 'Promised Land of sound health and happiness', towards everything good in life that you may wish or desire. Any easy and regular exercise will never disappoint no one trust me; you will always be the end winner! Just keep exercising; never give up in any situation or condition you may be!

MORE TIPS

To conceive and feel the abundances in life within and out of you, you must have known to often appreciate most of those things which give you pleasure; keep repeating your appreciation for them if and when you can; hold those things which give you deeper pleasure as sacred and as enough reason to live for the best possible. Keeping your life within such concept, stretching it out in time will proportionately replicate those pleasurable moments; and your reward shall be the nullification of all or most of the past bad moments you ever lived. In addition, the duct of happiness shall remain ajar!

-The above is the basic psychological processes to all forms of recurring or regenerating health which compliments mind and body for peace and harmony to foster!-

-It is wrong to do things for each other for money gain behind your mind; but absolutely and logically right to do things for each other for: love, passion or pleasure.

-Anything whatsoever, done with love, passion or pleasure, usually rekindles the flame of enthusiasm and soaring to the height of *burning-desires.*

-Enthusiasm unequivocally rewards with the highest degree of pleasure or pleasurable sensations in and out of entire created beings.

-Plain love, passion and pleasure, as intangibles as they maybe or seem, form the foundation of all human achievements; such subtle sensations when appreciated and retained to recur, speed the wheel of burning desire.

The sensation of burning desires in your hearts is the nucleus of any tangible human achievement; it is the engine of all feasible realizations

-Do your things with love and passion for the pleasure of doing so; so that the things that you chose to do, can truly be to your benefit!

The tangible value of a human's worth is the measure of the total average of good-deeds and seeds sown along the track of one's life.

Below is an excerpt from a book 'Good Health' by a renowned therapist Eugeni Evsikov from Siberia; published in one of the popular Weekly Newspapers in the Canary Island of Spain. I humbly practiced and found them unique and exceptional! Therefore, I immediately incorporated them for your benefit. I feel they are the best health practices I ever known! Enjoy!

ANCIENT CIVILIZATION GIVE MODERN-DAY RELIEF

The human body is very strong but the old methods of keeping it in good condition are not used enough.

One of these methods derives from Tibet where specialists recommend it for supporting the blood circulation and the immune, nervous and digestive systems. It is massage for the most important part of the body, releasing congestions and blockages and helping energy to flow along the meridian lines.

It is recommended that these exercises are done with the eyes closed; each one should be practiced five to ten times. Before starting, rub the hands together until they are warm.

-As soon as you awake, whilst still in bed, rub the ears up and down 30 times.

-Put the right hand over the forehead and the left one on top of the right hand. Massage the forehead head moving the hands from left to right, repeat 30 times then relax for a couple of minutes. This exercise is very effective for headaches, dizziness and circulation to the brain.

-**Massage the head** with the tips of the fingers starting from the forehead and moving down to the back of the head, then from the top of the head to the ears; do this 30 times. This will help blood circulation to the head; and will banish headaches, stress and tiredness.

-**With the eyes still closed**, use the thumbs to massage the eyes from the outer corner to the nose 15 times. This will help eyesight and the nervous system.

-**Put the right hand** on the throat and the left one over the right one, then move the hands down to the stomach 30 times – this improves the metabolism.

-**Put the right hand** on the stomach and the left one on the right hand, then move the hands from left to right 30 times, thus aiding the work of the digestive system.

-**Breathe in and out** from the stomach as hard as possible 30 times; this improves the activity of the liver, gall-bladder, the lymph system and the blood circulation.

-**Lie down, take the left leg** with both hands and pull it to the breast, repeat with the right leg then do both legs together, this helps the genital area and the stomach muscles.

-**Sit down, put the right leg** on the left knee and massage the foot 30 times; do the same with the left leg on the right knee. This exercise is effective for the whole body, as you press the reflexology points activating different systems, organs and glands in the body.

-**Put both hands** on the back of the neck, close the fingers together and pull the head down to the breast 30 times. This improves the blood circulation and helps dizziness and stiff necks.

-**Put the hands** on the ears, close them and press 30 times; this will improve tinnitus, headaches and the blood circulation to the head.

-**After doing these exercises,** drink two or three glasses of water and relax for five minutes. The best time to do all this is in the morning after waking up, before a meal or two hours afterwards.

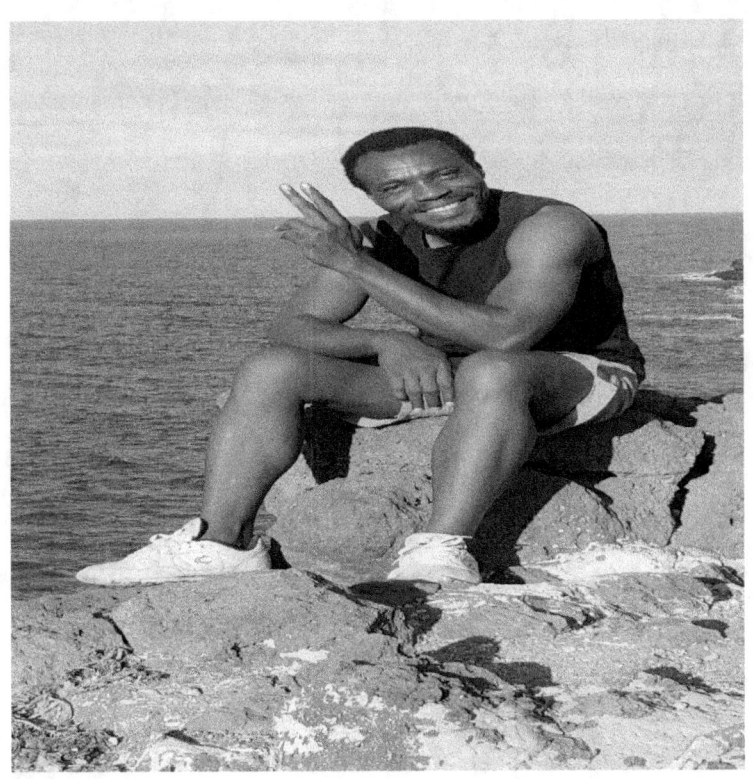

The Eight Universally Known Health Factors:

1. Always breathe fresh air

2. Drink plenty of water daily and shower regularly

3. Absorb enough sunshine each day

4. Eat well and healthy

5. Exercise regularly

6. Rest well regularly

7. Refrain from toxic substances

8. Always maintain positive thoughts

By practicing these eight factors of good health, it would put the organism in good conditions to face any harmful or infectious agent and, thus, the organisms can self-regenerate constantly without any issue.

FOOD AND FEEDING

-GOOD EATING HABIT FOR ALL CITIZENS-

Food is without doubt the life-giving substance; any material especially solid taken into the body and assimilated for purposes of growth, nourishment and ideas.

Food as air is next to life; no Food and Air, no life! To entire living creatures including humans,' food provides on daily basis to every one of them, all the energy they will need to activate the smooth functioning of their entire body organs for: moving, eating, talking, and working etc. No one can sustain life for long without food and water.

-Notwithstanding, many have adopted what we refer to as a 'bad eating habit' – eating at random without giving sufficient time for first food intake to go through complete digestion processes; and also, eating and indulging excessively. This kind of habit also hampers in most cases the real motive for food intake. It is note worthy for people to know and understand that, it is neither an obligation nor necessary to eat three square meals daily in order to remain healthy and happy.

-Food as for all other things of creation have their negative and positive sides; same food; as nice and as life-saving as they can be, happen to be amongst the top killer of people and animals. Most of the known diseases that usually attack humans come from food-intake; imagine the unfriendly odor of a rotten or spoilt food; your feces or excrement; the acidity in your urine; how devastating those can be! Therefore, good health and happy living is not about how much you eat but how well. As I said earlier, everything concerning life and humans, yield best results when done with discipline and in a balanced state of mind. Eventually, with self-discipline, in most cases some of us discover ways to eat correctly by adopting at will what we refer to as 'a good eating habit'.

A balanced person listens to the ways his/her body reacts to every food intake and unconsciously records the feelings he or she usually obtains after feeding on any thing; because everything that concerns humankind in relation to his growth is constantly noted or experienced through the aid of the intangibles known as 'feelings'.

-To actually eat healthy in accord with each ones private taste or 'gusto' there is the need to listen to the 'feel'; how you feel after eating whatever it is that you may eat. You should keep taking note of your favorite food intakes; relying on how your body system assimilates or rejects them. By so doing, with time you will accumulate a sound selection of food that your body system likes most and feels comfortable with.
When you are able to achieve that, you should then be able to allow those to be the food you will often be eating or feeding on most of the times.

-Never eat because others do eat or force yourself to eat at the time they do if your body will not be comfortable with the food at that moment; it is not wise to eat such things or at such times that will cause discomfort to your digestive systems.

-Do allow space and time in your stomach before pumping in more food. Eat only when you are hungry, not because there is food and it looks appetizing.

-Learn to eat very sparingly; always empty your bowels every morning before starting new food intakes and brush your teeth as many times as you may deem necessary.

-You should in reality brush your teeth and tongue each time you smell rotten food in your mouth and that should be as many times as is necessary- mostly whenever you eat any dairy products, chocolate and sugary things.

-Most people do not care much for their teeth and breath; they just eat, drink and smoke without maintaining the organs that make feeding possible – teeth, tongue and mouth as a whole should be the part of the body organs that should be treated with utmost respect and care plus the 'bowel cleansing' through a regular and daily excretion.

-Know that to eat healthy does not mean to eat more, worst of all is eating at random. -There is nothing unhealthier to the body than eating at all times- suffocating the metabolic system without allowing it adequate spacing to successfully finish its initial work of digestion.

-Eat a bit too much or too less for long, your body system will equally react negatively. Your main job as humans is to find the balance in any venture at all times.

Punctuality and regularity; those are some of the positive ingredients of entire universal life. Nature does not make much room for over-indulgence; over-indulgence weakens the soul and suffocates willpower.

-Every human that eats must as a matter of universal duty and obligation, be able to contribute in food production. Every human is supposed to produce their own food and shelter if all things remain equal; as in conformity with creational rules divested of manipulation and adulteration!

-Therefore, to regenerate your health the natural way, you have all the potentials and capabilities necessary to take control of your own health! What else have you without your health? You owe a duty to yourself to balance your spiritual and physical lifestyle. No one will do it for you without your consent or participation; because it is all there is for you in this entire world, your good health!

FEELING – what has mere feeling to do with wellness and fitness activities?
Feeling is the link between the unconscious, conscious and physical dimensions; the sensorial messenger whose duty is to deliver soul messages to the conscious counterpart whose own duty in turn is to deliver the message to the exterior dimension where the eyes can impress and categorize.

-When you make any form of exercise or do any activity whosoever, from such, a feeling is automatically registered, you may not notice these subtle natural reactions, but knowing them, being able to grasp the subtle messages from your unconscious or subconscious mind, is what brings harmony upon the physical. This is where wellness and fitness practices relate to feeling.

When you do something and your sensation from doing it registers pleasant, keep doing that, you feel good with the act. Your inner-self agrees, in harmony with your outside self.

-Strive to give most of your daily time to those things that make you feel good and well; you will long only feel good and quick to reject stress and unpleasant psychical and physical conditions.

- Listen to your heart and follow the good feelings of that silent voice staving from lack of adequate attention. Listen up to it and soon you will begin to do well in all things of interest to you. Your health will begin to regenerate the natural way!

-Learn to regenerate your only health the natural way following the desires and positive dictates of your unconscious and conscious soul. You will soon become a master of yourself and you will begin to appreciate the miracles of life, the beauty, the bliss and abundances of pain and joy. Savor and toast every moment without fear and doubts; only then will you begin to partake in the infinite wisdom of life!

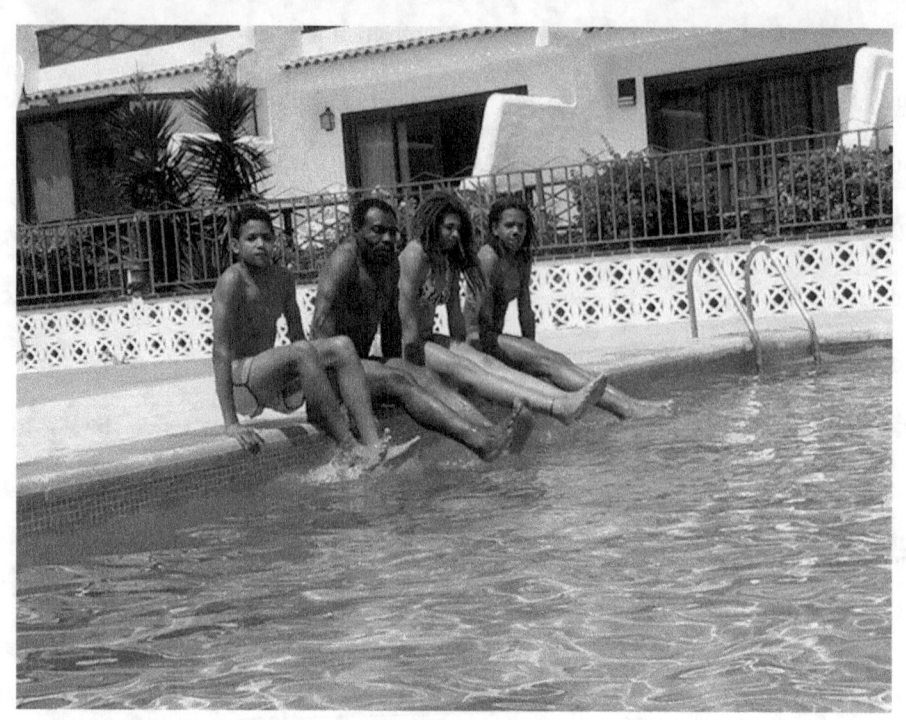

NEVER STOP TO DO THINGS; LIVING IS DOING AND DOING IS LIVING!

13- Drastic Measures for regenerating your health on day to day basis

1. Never drive to places you can walk without being too exhausted: walking or cycling to the place is healthier

2. Never work for money or for material gains behind your mind: work rather for your passion or for the love of what you are doing; that is healthier

3. Never stop to learn or to study; if you stop learning and studying your mind loses the power of regeneration. Things to learn and human ability to study are infinite; the more you know, the better you will live

4. Never overindulge in anything whatsoever in your life; little drops of water for long can make an ocean that can capsize mighty ships, destroy houses and drown people

5. Never give up respect for people, animals, and plants; when you respect people and things, in the same intensity peoples and things will give respect to you

6. Never stop to feel awe and amazement towards the Creator of all that is seen and unseen; never stop to ask, how did it all begin, and how did he make manifest all things?

7. Never stop to appreciate, admire and be thankful just for being alive and living

8. Delete as fast as you can anything whatsoever that stresses your mind in a negative way and in its place, replace it with those things that bring joy and peace to your innermost feelings

9. Never think first what you can get or gain out of anything that is worth doing; think first what value you can add to the place you are and to those people or things living around you. In a short time, everyone and everything around you will also, in equal intensity be thinking of what they can do to add value to your life. This is the only natural approach to acquire sound health and riches with peace and harmony

10. Never avoid anger; rather, learn to forgive and forget as soon as possible all that annoys you; make peace with those or things that annoy you. Your mind peace has no price whatsoever

11. Always think good thoughts from the deepest of your mind; with time, you can no more be provoked to anger and when you are, your anger will automatically be replaced by forgiveness and empathy

12. Exercise your body and mind every given day; do everything possible to carve time out for yourself to reflect or meditate. Your life is too precious and more important than any other thing on this awesome planet

13. Never keep or store anything whatsoever you do not really need; always satisfy only your immediate needs; or needs of this moment, now. Doing so will leave a room and enough energy to confront the next moment's needs when they manifest.

The above rules and regulations are very drastic and hard to abide by our present system. But, then, nature has its unfailing rules and regulations; between natures' rules and man-made rules, which of the two will you choose to obey?

Why are we always sick and weak and always in need? Is that the true nature of humanity? There are lots of things only you can discover for yourself; you have only but one life; take absolute care and control of it! That is all you owe to yourself and to your creator and to this world in general!

KNOW YOURSELF BETTER

Learn to be the sole manager of your wonderful life. Your mental attitude greatly influences your physical condition, actions and reactions both in public and in private. The personality of each person is determined by his or her regular actions and reactions on the entire affairs of life in general...

"How to Regenerate Your Failing Health" is not a normal book but rather, a simple and practical program meticulously structured to awaken the infinite capacities and potentials for positive deed found deep down within you

You will learn the importance of applying positive thinking when deciding and choosing on all the topics of the day and how to manage your holy-health and general well-being.

You will learn about yoga, its benefits and other combinations of exercises to increase your energy level necessary to balance your state of enthusiasm for living, working and being happy from day to day.

"How to Regenerate Your Failing Health" will deeply inspire you to take charge and control of your holy-health!